FIBROMYALGIA DIET COOKBOOK

Dr. Kimberly Carlos

Copyright © 2023 by Dr. Kimberly Carlos

TABLE OF CONTENT

INTRODUCTION

Once upon a time in a small town nestled among rolling hills, there lived a woman named Emma. She had battled fibromyalgia for years, enduring the constant pain, fatigue, and frustration that came with the condition. Doctors had offered little hope, prescribing medications that only provided temporary relief. Emma's life had become a relentless cycle of pain and despair.

One sunny morning, while browsing the internet for alternative treatments, Emma stumbled upon a blog post that caught her eye. It was written by Sarah, a woman who had successfully managed her fibromyalgia through dietary changes. Emma's curiosity was piqued, and she decided to delve deeper into Sarah's story.

Sarah had once been in a situation much like Emma's. She had suffered from fibromyalgia for years until she decided to take matters into her own hands. She began researching and experimenting with her diet, eventually discovering a combination of whole foods that drastically improved her condition.

Emma decided to follow in Sarah's footsteps. She started by eliminating processed foods, sugar, and gluten from her diet. Instead, she focused on eating plenty of fruits, vegetables, lean proteins, and healthy fats. She also incorporated anti-inflammatory foods like turmeric and ginger into her meals.

Weeks turned into months, and Emma's dedication to her new diet paid off. She began to notice a significant reduction in her pain and fatigue. She had more energy to do the things she loved, like gardening and spending time with her grandchildren. Slowly but steadily, her fibromyalgia symptoms diminished, and her quality of life improved.

Emma couldn't believe the transformation. She reached out to Sarah, thanking her for sharing her story and guiding her toward this newfound freedom from pain. Emma's journey to healing wasn't easy, but it was a testament to the power of the right diet and the determination to regain control of one's life.

As the years passed, Emma continued to thrive, proving that with the right approach, even the most stubborn of ailments could be conquered. Her story served as an inspiration to others facing similar challenges, offering hope that a brighter, pain-free future was within reach for anyone willing to take that first step toward dietary change.

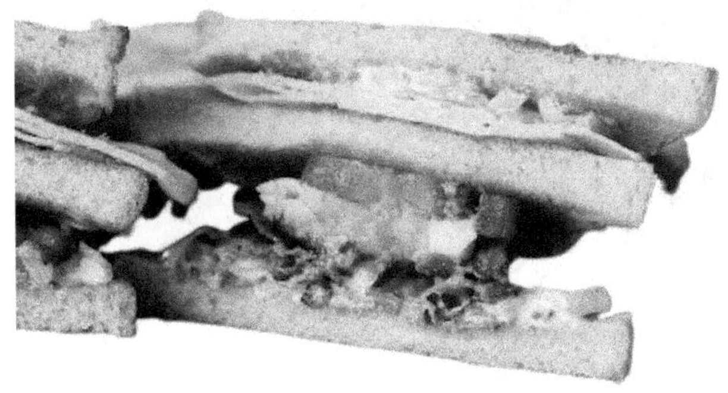

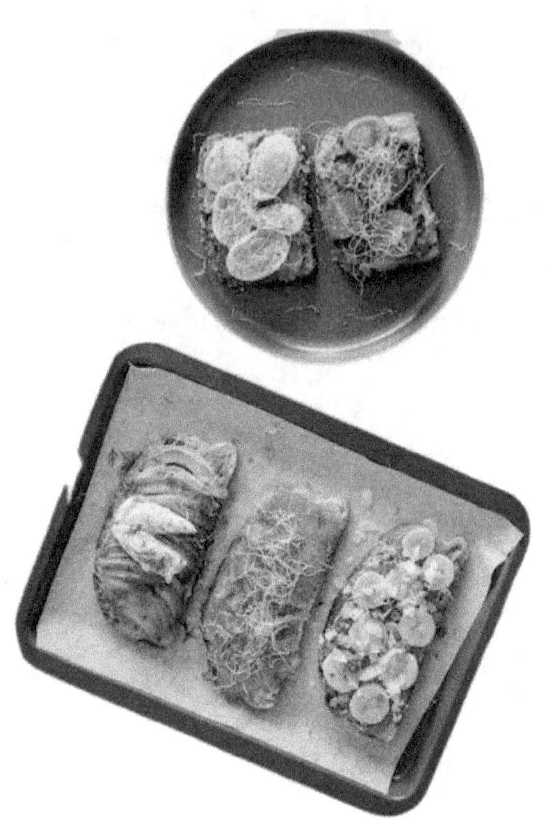

CHAPTER ONE

Fibromyalgia: Types, Causes and Symptoms

Fibromyalgia is a complex and often misunderstood medical condition that primarily affects the musculoskeletal system. It is characterized by widespread, chronic pain, along with a range of other symptoms. While the exact cause of fibromyalgia remains unknown, researchers have identified several potential factors that contribute to its development.

Here, we'll explore the different types, causes, and symptoms of fibromyalgia:

Types of Fibromyalgia

1. Primary Fibromyalgia: This is the most common type of fibromyalgia, where the condition occurs without any underlying medical conditions or specific triggers.

2. Secondary Fibromyalgia: Secondary fibromyalgia is associated with other medical conditions, such as rheumatoid arthritis, lupus, or osteoarthritis. It tends to develop as a result of these underlying conditions.

Causes of Fibromyalgia

1. Genetic Predisposition: While not directly inherited, there appears to be a genetic component to fibromyalgia. Individuals with a family history of the condition may be more prone to developing it.

2. Abnormal Pain Processing: Fibromyalgia is thought to involve abnormalities in how the brain and spinal cord process pain signals. This can lead to an increased perception of pain.

3. Physical Trauma or Injury: Some cases of fibromyalgia are triggered by physical trauma, such as car accidents or injuries, which can amplify pain sensations.

4. Infections and Illnesses: Certain infections and illnesses can increase the risk of fibromyalgia, as they may trigger or exacerbate symptoms. These can include viral infections or surgeries.

Common Symptoms of Fibromyalgia

1. Widespread Pain: The hallmark symptom of fibromyalgia is widespread, chronic pain that affects multiple areas of the body. It often involves tender points, where pressure can cause increased discomfort.

2. Fatigue: Individuals with fibromyalgia frequently experience overwhelming fatigue, even after a full night's sleep. This fatigue can be debilitating and affect daily activities.

3. Sleep Disturbances: Sleep disorders, such as restless leg syndrome or sleep apnea, are common among fibromyalgia patients. These issues contribute to the persistent fatigue.

4. Cognitive Symptoms (Fibro Fog): Many people with fibromyalgia report cognitive difficulties, often referred to as "fibro fog." This includes memory problems, difficulty concentrating, and mental confusion.

5. Stiffness: Morning stiffness and muscle stiffness are common symptoms of fibromyalgia, making it challenging to move and perform everyday tasks.

6. Headaches: Chronic headaches, including tension-type and migraines, are prevalent in fibromyalgia sufferers.

7. Irritable Bowel Syndrome (IBS): Some individuals with fibromyalgia also experience gastrointestinal symptoms, such as abdominal pain, bloating, and altered bowel habits.

8. Depression and Anxiety: Fibromyalgia can have a significant impact on mental health, often leading to depression and anxiety due to the constant pain and limitations it imposes.

9. Sensitivity to External Stimuli: Heightened sensitivity to light, noise, temperature, and odors is common in fibromyalgia patients.

Understanding the different types, potential causes, and wide-ranging symptoms of fibromyalgia is essential for early diagnosis and effective management. Since fibromyalgia is a chronic condition, a multidisciplinary approach involving healthcare providers, lifestyle modifications, and, in some cases, medication, can help individuals manage their symptoms and improve their quality of life.

Following a Fibromyalgia Diet with Benefits

Following a fibromyalgia diet can help manage the symptoms of this condition and improve overall well-being. While there's no one-size-fits-all approach, as dietary needs vary from person to person, these are some general guidelines to help you get started on a fibromyalgia-friendly diet:

1. Balance Your Diet: Aim for a balanced diet that includes a variety of whole foods. Focus on fruits, vegetables, lean proteins, whole grains, and healthy fats. This provides essential nutrients and helps maintain stable energy levels.

2. Hydration: Drink plenty of water throughout the day to stay hydrated. Dehydration can worsen fibromyalgia symptoms.

3. Limit Processed Foods: Reduce or eliminate processed foods, which often contain additives, preservatives, and artificial ingredients that can exacerbate symptoms.

4. Avoid Trigger Foods: Identify and avoid foods that may trigger or worsen your symptoms. Common culprits include caffeine, alcohol, sugar, and certain artificial sweeteners. Keep a food diary to track how specific foods affect you.

5. Choose Anti-Inflammatory Foods: Incorporate foods with anti-inflammatory properties into your diet, such as fatty fish (e.g., salmon), turmeric, ginger, and foods rich in antioxidants (berries, leafy greens).

6. Include Omega-3 Fatty Acids: Omega-3 fatty acids, found in fish, flaxseeds, and walnuts, can help reduce inflammation and alleviate pain associated with **fibromyalgia.**

7. Balanced Carbohydrates: Opt for complex carbohydrates like whole grains (brown rice, quinoa, oats) to provide sustained energy and help stabilize blood sugar levels.

8. Adequate Protein: Ensure you're getting enough protein from sources like lean meats, poultry, fish, legumes, and tofu to support muscle health.

9. Small, Frequent Meals: Instead of three large meals, consider eating smaller, more frequent meals to prevent energy crashes and maintain steady blood sugar levels.

10. Consider Supplements: Consult your healthcare provider about supplement options that may benefit fibromyalgia patients, such as magnesium, vitamin D, and coenzyme Q10. However, it's essential to get professional advice before taking any supplements.

11. Mindful Eating: Practice mindful eating by savoring each bite, eating slowly, and paying attention to your body's hunger and fullness cues.

12. Monitor Triggers: Keep a food diary to track your diet and symptoms. This can help you identify specific foods or patterns that exacerbate your fibromyalgia symptoms.

13. Stay Consistent: Consistency is key when following a fibromyalgia diet. Stick to your chosen dietary plan and give it time to see if it helps manage your symptoms.

14. Seek Professional Guidance: Consider working with a registered dietitian or nutritionist who specializes in fibromyalgia to create a personalized diet plan tailored to your specific needs.

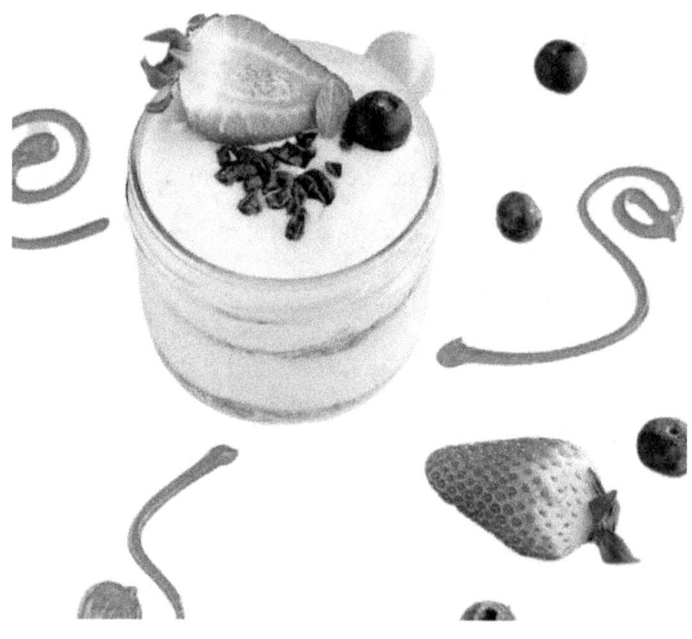

CHAPTER TWO

14-Day Fibromyalgia Diet Meal Plan

Day 1

- Breakfast: Greek yogurt with berries and a sprinkle of ground flaxseeds.
- Snack: Carrot and cucumber sticks with hummus.
- Lunch: Grilled chicken breast with quinoa and steamed broccoli.
- Snack: A small handful of almonds.
- Dinner: Baked salmon with asparagus and a side salad.

Day 2

- Breakfast: Oatmeal with sliced bananas and a drizzle of honey.
- Snack: Apple slices with almond butter.
- Lunch: Lentil soup and a mixed greens salad with balsamic vinaigrette.
- Snack: Greek yogurt with honey and a handful of walnuts.
- Dinner: Baked chicken thighs with roasted sweet potatoes and Brussels sprouts.

Day 3

- Breakfast: Spinach and mushroom omelet with whole-grain toast.
- Snack: Celery sticks with peanut butter.
- Lunch: Quinoa salad with chickpeas, cucumber, and feta cheese.
- Snack: Mixed berries and a small piece of dark chocolate.
- Dinner: Grilled shrimp with quinoa and steamed spinach.

Day 4

- Breakfast: Smoothie with spinach, banana, almond milk, and a scoop of protein powder.
- Snack: Cottage cheese with pineapple chunks.
- Lunch: Turkey and avocado wrap with a side of mixed greens.
- Snack: Sliced pear with a sprinkle of cinnamon.
- Dinner: Baked cod with a side of brown rice and sautéed zucchini.

Day 5

- Breakfast: Overnight oats made with rolled oats, chia seeds, almond milk, and topped with sliced strawberries.
- Snack: A small handful of cashews.
- Lunch: Quinoa and black bean stuffed bell peppers.
- Snack: Sliced cucumber with tzatziki sauce.
- Dinner: Grilled chicken breast with quinoa and roasted carrots.

Day 6

- Breakfast: Scrambled eggs with spinach, tomatoes, and a slice of whole-grain toast.
- Snack: Sliced bell peppers with guacamole.
- Lunch: Salmon salad with mixed greens, cherry tomatoes, and a lemon vinaigrette.
- Snack: Sliced mango.
- Dinner: Baked turkey meatballs with spaghetti squash and marinara sauce.

Day 7

- Breakfast: Smoothie with kale, pineapple, Greek yogurt, and a spoonful of flaxseeds.
- Snack: A small handful of sunflower seeds.
- Lunch: Lentil and vegetable stir-fry with brown rice.
- Snack: Sliced kiwi.
- Dinner: Baked tilapia with quinoa and steamed green beans.

Day 8

- Breakfast: Overnight chia seed pudding with almond milk, topped with sliced peaches and a sprinkle of cinnamon.
- Snack: Baby carrots with tzatziki sauce.
- Lunch: Turkey and vegetable stir-fry with brown rice.
- Snack: Sliced strawberries with a dollop of Greek yogurt.
- Dinner: Baked chicken breast with quinoa and steamed broccoli.

Day 9

- Breakfast: Scrambled eggs with spinach and feta cheese, served with a side of sliced oranges.
- Snack: A small handful of trail mix (nuts and dried fruits).
- Lunch: Spinach and kale salad with grilled shrimp, cherry tomatoes, and a lemon-tahini dressing.
- Snack: Sliced apple with a drizzle of honey.
- Dinner: Baked cod with a side of couscous and roasted asparagus.

Day 10

- Breakfast: Whole-grain pancakes topped with Greek yogurt and fresh berries.
- Snack: Sliced bell peppers with hummus.
- Lunch: Quinoa and black bean bowl with avocado, corn, and salsa.
- Snack: Sliced kiwi and a few almonds.
- Dinner: Baked turkey breast with quinoa and sautéed spinach.

Day 11

- Breakfast: Smoothie with banana, spinach, almond milk, and a scoop of protein powder.
- Snack: Sliced cucumber with tzatziki sauce.
- Lunch: Lentil soup with a mixed greens salad and vinaigrette.
- Snack: A small handful of cashews.
- Dinner: Grilled chicken thighs with brown rice and steamed Brussels sprouts.

Day 12

- Breakfast: Omelet with mushrooms, onions, and bell peppers, served with a slice of whole-grain toast.
- Snack: Sliced pear with almond butter.
- Lunch: Tuna salad with mixed greens and a lemon-tahini dressing.
- Snack: Greek yogurt with honey and a sprinkle of granola.
- Dinner: Baked salmon with quinoa and roasted carrots.

Day 13

- Breakfast: Whole-grain waffles topped with sliced strawberries and a dollop of Greek yogurt.
- Snack: Baby carrots with hummus.
- Lunch: Chicken and vegetable curry with brown rice.
- Snack: Sliced mango.
- Dinner: Grilled shrimp with quinoa and sautéed zucchini.

Day 14

- Breakfast: Smoothie with blueberries, kale, Greek yogurt, and a spoonful of flaxseeds.
- Snack: A small handful of sunflower seeds.
- Lunch: Quinoa and vegetable-stuffed bell peppers.
- Snack: Sliced oranges.
- Dinner: Baked chicken breast with brown rice and steamed green beans.

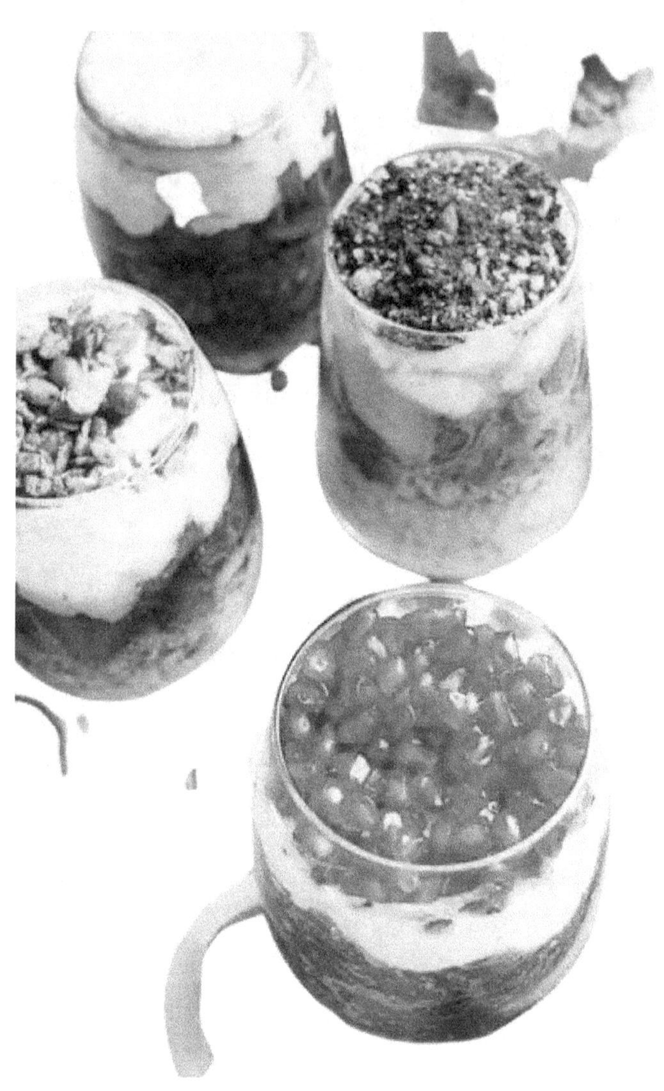

CHAPTER THREE

Fibromyalgia Diet Breakfast Recipes

Breakfast is an essential part of the day, especially for those managing fibromyalgia. It provides much-needed energy and nutrients to kickstart your morning while considering dietary choices that can help alleviate symptoms. Here are 10 fibromyalgia-friendly breakfast recipes to add variety and flavor to your morning routine.

1. Blueberry Almond Smoothie Bowl

Ingredients:

- 1 cup frozen blueberries
- 1 ripe banana
- 1/4 cup almond milk
- 1/4 cup Greek yogurt
- 1 tbsp almond butter
- Toppings: sliced almonds, fresh blueberries, honey (optional)

Instructions:

1. Blend blueberries, banana, almond milk, Greek yogurt, and almond butter until smooth.

2. Pour into a bowl and top with sliced almonds, fresh blueberries, and a drizzle of honey if desired.

3. Enjoy!

Cooking Time: 5 minutes

2. Spinach and Mushroom Omelet

Ingredients:

- 2 eggs
- 1/4 cup chopped spinach
- 1/4 cup sliced mushrooms
- 2 tbsp grated Parmesan cheese
- Salt and pepper to taste

Instructions:

1. Whisk eggs in a bowl and season with salt and pepper.

2. Heat a non-stick skillet over medium heat and add chopped spinach and mushrooms.

3. Pour the whisked eggs over the vegetables.

4. Sprinkle Parmesan cheese over the top.

5. Cook until set, then fold the omelet in half.

6. Serve hot.

Cooking Time: 10 minutes

3. Quinoa Breakfast Bowl

Ingredients:

- 1/2 cup cooked quinoa
- 1/4 cup sliced strawberries
- 1/4 cup chopped nuts (e.g., almonds, walnuts)
- 1/4 cup Greek yogurt
- Drizzle of honey (optional)

Instructions:

1. Place cooked quinoa in a bowl.

2. Top with sliced strawberries, chopped nuts, and Greek yogurt.

3. Drizzle with honey if desired.

4. Mix and enjoy!

Cooking Time: 5 minutes (if quinoa is pre-cooked)

4. Peanut Butter and Banana Toast

Ingredients:

- 1 slice of whole-grain bread
- 2 tbsp peanut butter
- 1/2 ripe banana, sliced
- Drizzle of honey (optional)

Instructions:

1. Toast the bread to your preferred level of crispiness.

2. Spread peanut butter on the toast.

3. Top with banana slices.

4. Drizzle with honey if desired.

Cooking Time: 5 minutes

5. Greek Yogurt Parfait

Ingredients:

- 1/2 cup Greek yogurt
- 1/4 cup granola
- 1/4 cup mixed berries (e.g., strawberries, blueberries)
- Drizzle of honey (optional)

Instructions:

1. In a glass or bowl, layer Greek yogurt, granola, and mixed berries.

2. Drizzle with honey if desired.

3. Repeat layers if desired.

4. Serve chilled.

Cooking Time: 5 minutes

6. Chia Seed Pudding

Ingredients:

- 2 tbsp chia seeds
- 1/2 cup almond milk
- 1/4 tsp vanilla extract
- Sliced kiwi and berries for topping

Instructions:

1. Mix chia seeds, almond milk, and vanilla extract in a jar or bowl.

2. Refrigerate overnight or for at least 2 hours until it thickens.

3. Top with sliced kiwi and berries before serving.

Cooking Time: 2 hours (mostly inactive)

7. Scrambled Tofu with Veggies

Ingredients:

- 1/2 cup crumbled tofu
- 1/4 cup diced bell peppers
- 1/4 cup diced onions

- 1/4 cup diced tomatoes
- 1/4 tsp turmeric
- Salt and pepper to taste

Instructions:

1. Heat a skillet over medium heat and sauté onions and bell peppers until softened.

2. Add crumbled tofu, diced tomatoes, turmeric, salt, and pepper.

3. Cook until tofu is heated through.

4. Serve hot.

Cooking Time: 10 minutes

8. Banana and Walnut Muffins (Gluten-free)

Ingredients:

- 2 ripe bananas, mashed
- 1/4 cup almond flour
- 1/4 cup coconut flour
- 1/4 cup chopped walnuts
- 1/4 cup honey or maple syrup

- 2 eggs
- 1/2 tsp baking soda
- 1/2 tsp vanilla extract
- Pinch of salt

Instructions:

1. Preheat the oven to 350°F (175°C) and line a muffin tin with paper liners.

2. In a bowl, mix mashed bananas, almond flour, coconut flour, chopped walnuts, honey or maple syrup, eggs, baking soda, vanilla extract, and a pinch of salt until well combined.

3. Spoon the batter into muffin cups, filling each about 2/3 full.

4. Bake for 20-25 minutes or until a toothpick comes out clean.

5. Allow to cool before serving.

Cooking Time: 25 minutes

9. Avocado and Tomato Toast

Ingredients:

- 1 slice of whole-grain bread
- 1/2 ripe avocado, mashed
- Sliced cherry tomatoes
- Fresh basil leaves
- Salt and pepper to taste

Instructions:

1. Toast the bread to your preferred level of crispiness.

2. Spread mashed avocado on the toast.

3. Top with sliced cherry tomatoes and fresh basil.

4. Season with salt and pepper.

Cooking Time: 5 minutes

10. Sweet Potato Breakfast Hash

Ingredients:

- 1 small sweet potato, peeled and diced
- 1/4 cup diced red bell pepper
- 1/4 cup diced onion

- 1/4 cup diced zucchini
- 2 eggs
- Olive oil for cooking
- Salt and pepper to taste

Instructions:

1. Heat olive oil in a skillet over medium heat.

2. Add diced sweet potato and cook until slightly tender.

3. Add diced red bell pepper, onion, and zucchini. Cook until all vegetables are tender.

4. Push the vegetables to one side of the skillet and crack the eggs into the other side.

5. Cook the eggs until the whites are set but the yolks are still runny.

6. Serve the eggs over the sweet potato and vegetable hash.

7. Season with salt and pepper.

Cooking Time: 15 minutes

Fibromyalgia Diet Lunch Recipes

1. Quinoa and Black Bean Salad

This quinoa and black bean salad is packed with protein and fiber to keep you full and energized throughout the day.

Ingredients:

- 1 cup cooked quinoa
- 1 can (15 oz) black beans, drained and rinsed
- 1 cup diced bell peppers (various colors)
- 1 cup corn kernels (fresh or frozen)
- 1/4 cup chopped fresh cilantro
- Juice of 1 lime
- Salt and pepper to taste

Instructions:

1. In a large bowl, combine cooked quinoa, black beans, diced bell peppers, corn, and cilantro.

2. Squeeze the lime juice over the salad and season with salt and pepper.

3. Toss well and refrigerate until ready to serve.

Cooking Time: 15 minutes (if quinoa is pre-cooked)

2. Mediterranean Chickpea Salad

This Mediterranean-inspired salad is full of fresh ingredients and Mediterranean flavors.

Ingredients:

- 1 can (15 oz) chickpeas, drained and rinsed
- 1 cup diced cucumber
- 1 cup cherry tomatoes, halved
- 1/4 cup diced red onion
- 1/4 cup chopped fresh parsley
- Feta cheese (optional)
- Lemon juice and olive oil for dressing
- Salt and pepper to taste

Instructions:

1. In a large bowl, combine chickpeas, diced cucumber, cherry tomatoes, red onion, and parsley.

2. Drizzle with lemon juice and olive oil and season with salt and pepper.

3. Top with crumbled feta cheese if desired.

4. Chill before serving.

3. Spinach and Strawberry Salad

This refreshing salad combines the sweetness of strawberries with the freshness of spinach and a tangy vinaigrette.

Ingredients:

- 2 cups fresh baby spinach
- 1 cup sliced strawberries
- 1/4 cup sliced almonds
- 1/4 cup crumbled goat cheese (optional)
- Balsamic vinaigrette dressing

Instructions:

1. In a salad bowl, combine fresh baby spinach, sliced strawberries, and sliced almonds.

2. Top with crumbled goat cheese if desired.

3. Drizzle with balsamic vinaigrette dressing before serving.

Cooking Time: 10 minutes

4. Lentil and Vegetable Soup

A hearty and nutritious lentil soup that's easy to make and perfect for those with fibromyalgia.

Ingredients:

- 1 cup dried green or brown lentils, rinsed and drained
- 1 cup diced carrots
- 1 cup diced celery
- 1 cup diced onions
- 4 cups vegetable or chicken broth
- 1 tsp dried thyme
- Salt and pepper to taste

Instructions:

1. In a large pot, sauté onions, carrots, and celery until slightly softened.

2. Add lentils, broth, dried thyme, salt, and pepper.

3. Bring to a boil, then reduce heat and simmer for about 20-25 minutes until lentils are tender.

4. Adjust seasoning as needed and serve hot.

Cooking Time: 30 minutes

5. Grilled Chicken and Vegetable Wrap

This grilled chicken and vegetable wrap is a satisfying and nutritious lunch option.

Ingredients:

- 1 boneless, skinless chicken breast
- 1 whole-grain tortilla
- 1/2 cup mixed greens
- Sliced tomatoes, cucumbers, and red bell peppers
- Hummus or Greek yogurt dressing

Instructions:

1. Season the chicken breast with your preferred seasonings.

2. Grill the chicken until cooked through, then slice it into strips.

3. Lay out the whole-grain tortilla and spread a layer of hummus or Greek yogurt dressing.

4. Add mixed greens, sliced chicken, and your choice of vegetables.

5. Roll up the tortilla and enjoy.

Cooking Time: 15-20 minutes

6. Sweet Potato and Chickpea Curry

This hearty curry combines the creaminess of sweet potatoes with the protein of chickpeas.

Ingredients:

- 1 large sweet potato, peeled and diced
- 1 can (15 oz) chickpeas, drained and rinsed
- 1 cup diced tomatoes
- 1 cup coconut milk
- 1 tbsp curry powder
- Salt and pepper to taste
- Fresh cilantro for garnish (optional)

Instructions:

1. In a large skillet, combine sweet potato, chickpeas, diced tomatoes, and coconut milk.

2. Stir in curry powder, salt, and pepper.

3. Simmer over medium heat until sweet potatoes are tender and the curry has thickened.

4. Serve hot, garnished with fresh cilantro if desired.

Cooking Time: 25 minutes

7. Salmon and Avocado Salad

A protein-packed salad featuring salmon and avocado for a satisfying and nutritious lunch.

Ingredients:

- 4 oz grilled or baked salmon fillet, flaked
- 1/2 avocado, sliced
- 2 cups mixed greens
- Cherry tomatoes, halved
- Balsamic vinaigrette dressing

Instructions:

1. Arrange mixed greens on a plate.

2. Top with flaked salmon, sliced avocado, and cherry tomato halves.

3. Drizzle with balsamic vinaigrette dressing.

4. Enjoy your salmon and avocado salad.

Cooking Time: 15 minutes (if salmon is pre-cooked)

8. Quinoa and Vegetable Stir-Fry

A quick and healthy quinoa stir-fry packed with colorful vegetables.

Ingredients:

- 1 cup cooked quinoa
- 1 cup mixed vegetables (e.g., bell peppers, broccoli, carrots)
- 1/4 cup diced onion
- 2 cloves garlic, minced
- Low-sodium soy sauce or stir-fry sauce
- Olive oil for cooking

Instructions:

1. Heat olive oil in a large skillet or wok.

2. Sauté diced onion and minced garlic until fragrant.

3. Add mixed vegetables and stir-fry until tender-crisp.

4. Stir in cooked quinoa and a splash of low-sodium soy sauce or stir-fry sauce.

5. Cook for a few more minutes until heated through.

6. Serve hot.

Cooking Time: 15 minutes (if quinoa is pre-cooked)

9. Tomato Basil Soup

A comforting and classic tomato basil soup recipe that's perfect for a soothing lunch.

Ingredients:

- 1 can (28 oz) crushed tomatoes
- 1/4 cup fresh basil leaves
- 1/4 cup diced onion
- 1 clove garlic, minced
- 2 cups vegetable broth
- 1/2 cup coconut milk (or dairy-free milk of choice)
- Salt and pepper to taste

Instructions:

1. In a large pot, sauté diced onion and minced garlic until softened.

2. Add crushed tomatoes and vegetable broth.

3. Bring to a boil, then reduce heat and simmer for about 10 minutes.

4. Stir in fresh basil leaves and coconut milk.

5. Use an immersion blender to blend the soup until smooth.

6. Season with salt and pepper to taste.

7. Serve hot.

Cooking Time: 20 minutes

10. Turkey and Avocado Wrap

A protein-packed wrap with lean turkey and creamy avocado for a satisfying and nutritious lunch.

Ingredients:

- 4 oz sliced turkey breast
- 1 whole-grain tortilla
- 1/2 ripe avocado, sliced
- Mixed greens
- Sliced bell peppers
- Dijon mustard or Greek yogurt dressing

Instructions:

1. Lay out the whole-grain tortilla and spread a layer of Dijon mustard or Greek yogurt dressing.

2. Add mixed greens, sliced turkey, avocado, and bell peppers.

3. Roll up the tortilla and enjoy your turkey and avocado wrap.

Cooking Time: 10 minutes (if turkey is pre-cooked)

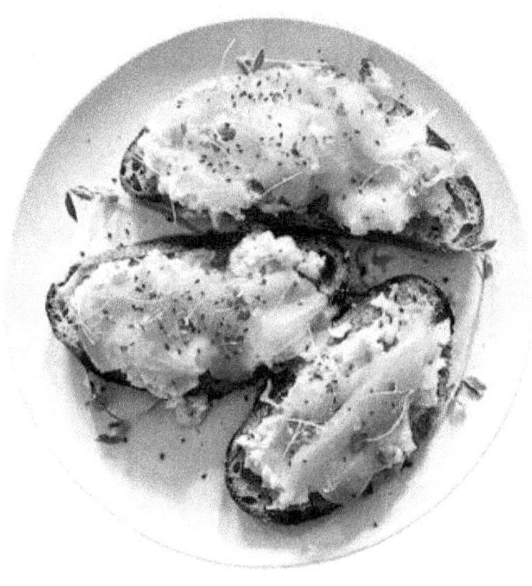

CHAPTER FOUR

Fibromyalgia Diet Dinner Recipes

1. Lemon Garlic Baked Chicken

This simple, flavorful baked chicken is easy on the stomach and perfect for a fibromyalgia-friendly dinner.

Ingredients:

- 4 boneless, skinless chicken breasts
- Juice of 1 lemon
- 3 cloves garlic, minced
- 2 tbsp olive oil
- 1 tsp dried oregano
- Salt and pepper to taste

Instructions:

1. Preheat your oven to 375°F (190°C).

2. In a small bowl, combine lemon juice, minced garlic, olive oil, dried oregano, salt, and pepper.

3. Place chicken breasts in a baking dish and pour the lemon-garlic mixture over them.

4. Bake for 25-30 minutes or until the chicken is cooked through.

Cooking Time: 30 minutes

2. Roasted Vegetable and Quinoa Bowl

A wholesome bowl filled with roasted vegetables and quinoa, providing a balanced and nutritious dinner.

Ingredients:

- 1 cup cooked quinoa
- Assorted vegetables (e.g., bell peppers, zucchini, carrots)
- Olive oil
- Herbs (e.g., thyme, rosemary)
- Salt and pepper
- Balsamic glaze (optional)

Instructions:

1. Preheat your oven to 425°F (220°C).

2. Toss chopped vegetables with olive oil, herbs, salt, and pepper.

3. Roast in the oven for about 20-25 minutes until tender and slightly caramelized.

4. Serve the roasted vegetables over a bed of cooked quinoa.

5. Drizzle with balsamic glaze if desired.

Cooking Time: 30 minutes

3. Salmon with Dill Sauce

Salmon is rich in omega-3 fatty acids, which may help reduce inflammation associated with fibromyalgia.

Ingredients:

- 4 salmon fillets
- 1/4 cup Greek yogurt
- 1 tbsp fresh dill, chopped
- Juice of 1/2 lemon
- Salt and pepper to taste

Instructions:

1. Preheat your oven to 375°F (190°C).

2. Season salmon fillets with salt and pepper and place them on a baking sheet.

3. Bake for 15-20 minutes or until the salmon flakes easily with a fork.

4. While the salmon is baking, mix Greek yogurt, fresh dill, and lemon juice in a bowl.

5. Serve the salmon with a dollop of the dill sauce.

Cooking Time: 20 minutes

4. Vegetable and Lentil Curry

A comforting and flavorful vegetable and lentil curry that's rich in fiber and plant-based protein.

Ingredients:

- 1 cup dried red lentils, rinsed and drained
- Assorted vegetables (e.g., bell peppers, cauliflower, peas)
- 1 can (15 oz) diced tomatoes
- 1 can (13.5 oz) coconut milk
- 2 tbsp curry powder
- Salt and pepper to taste
- Olive oil for cooking

Instructions:

1. In a large pot, sauté assorted vegetables in olive oil until slightly tender.

2. Add dried red lentils, diced tomatoes, coconut milk, curry powder, salt, and pepper.

3. Simmer for about 20-25 minutes until lentils are cooked and vegetables are tender.

4. Adjust seasoning as needed and serve hot.

Cooking Time: 30 minutes

5. Lemon Garlic Shrimp Pasta (Gluten-free)

A gluten-free pasta dish featuring shrimp, fresh lemon, and garlic for a zesty and satisfying dinner.

Ingredients:

- 8 oz gluten-free pasta (e.g., brown rice or chickpea pasta)
- 1 lb large shrimp, peeled and deveined
- 3 cloves garlic, minced
- Juice of 2 lemons

-   2 tbsp olive oil

-   Fresh parsley for garnish (optional)

-   Salt and pepper to taste

Instructions:

1. Cook the gluten-free pasta according to package instructions.

2. While the pasta is cooking, heat olive oil in a large skillet over medium-high heat.

3. Add minced garlic and shrimp, cooking for 2-3 minutes on each side until they turn pink.

4. Drain cooked pasta and toss it with lemon juice, salt, and pepper.

5. Serve the shrimp over the lemon garlic pasta.

6. Garnish with fresh parsley if desired.

Cooking Time: 20 minutes

6. Baked Turkey Meatballs with Zoodles

A light and healthy dinner featuring baked turkey meatballs served over zucchini noodles (zoodles).

Ingredients:

- 1 lb ground turkey
- 1/4 cup almond meal (or gluten-free breadcrumbs)
- 1/4 cup grated Parmesan cheese (optional)
- 1 egg
- 1 clove garlic, minced
- Salt and pepper to taste
- 4 medium zucchinis, spiralized into zoodles
- Marinara sauce

Instructions:

1. Preheat your oven to 375°F (190°C).

2. In a bowl, mix ground turkey, almond meal, Parmesan cheese, egg, minced garlic, salt, and pepper.

3. Form the mixture into meatballs and place them on a baking sheet.

4. Bake for 20-25 minutes until meatballs are cooked

through.

5. In a separate pan, sauté zucchini noodles with marinara sauce until heated.

6. Serve the turkey meatballs over the zoodles.

 Cooking Time: 30 minutes

7. Vegetarian Stir-Fried Tofu and Broccoli

A vegetarian stir-fry featuring tofu and broccoli for a quick and nutritious dinner option.

Ingredients:

- 14 oz firm tofu, cubed
- 2 cups broccoli florets
- 2 cloves garlic, minced
- 2 tbsp low-sodium soy sauce
- 1 tbsp sesame oil
- Red pepper flakes (optional)
- Olive oil for cooking
- Cooked brown rice (optional)

Instructions:

1. Heat olive oil in a large skillet or wok over medium-high heat.

2. Add minced garlic and cubed tofu, stir-frying until tofu is golden.

3. Add broccoli florets and continue to stir-fry for a few minutes.

4. Pour in low-sodium soy sauce, sesame oil, and red pepper flakes if desired.

5. Continue to stir-fry until the broccoli is tender and the tofu is coated with the sauce.

6. Serve as is or over cooked brown rice if preferred.

Cooking Time: 20 minutes

8. Baked Cod with Herbed Quinoa

A light and healthy dinner featuring baked cod and herbed quinoa for a satisfying and nutritious meal.

Ingredients:

- 4 cod fillets
- 1 cup quinoa, rinsed and drained
- 2 cups vegetable broth
- Fresh herbs (e.g., parsley, dill, chives)
- Olive oil
- Lemon wedges for serving
- Salt and pepper to taste

Instructions:

1. Preheat your oven to 375°F (190°C).

2. Season cod fillets with olive oil, fresh herbs, salt, and pepper.

3. Place cod fillets on a baking sheet and bake for 15-20 minutes or until the fish flakes easily with a fork.

4. While the cod is baking, bring vegetable broth to a boil in a pot.

5. Add quinoa, reduce heat, and simmer for about 15 minutes or until quinoa is cooked and liquid is absorbed.

6. Fluff the quinoa with a fork and stir in additional fresh

herbs.

7. Serve baked cod over herbed quinoa with lemon wedges.

Cooking Time: 30 minutes

9. Sweet Potato and Chickpea Curry (Vegetarian)

A comforting and flavorful vegetarian curry featuring sweet potatoes and chickpeas.

Ingredients:

- 2 large sweet potatoes, peeled and diced
- 1 can (15 oz) chickpeas, drained and rinsed
- 1 can (13.5 oz) coconut milk
- 1 tbsp curry powder
- 2 cloves garlic, minced
- Olive oil for cooking
- Salt and pepper to taste

Instructions:

1. In a large pot, sauté minced garlic in olive oil until fragrant.

2. Add diced sweet potatoes and chickpeas.

3. Stir in curry powder, salt, and pepper.

4. Pour in coconut milk and simmer for about 20-25 minutes until sweet potatoes are tender.

5. Adjust seasoning as needed and serve hot.

Cooking Time: 30 minutes

10. Grilled Turkey Burgers with Sweet Potato Fries

A fibromyalgia-friendly twist on a classic burger and fries, using lean turkey and sweet potato fries.

Ingredients:

- 1 lb ground turkey
- Whole-grain burger buns or lettuce wraps
- Sliced tomatoes, lettuce, and onions
- 2 large sweet potatoes, cut into fries
- Olive oil
- Paprika, garlic powder, and salt for seasoning
- Cooking spray

Instructions:

1. Preheat your grill to medium-high heat.

2. Form ground turkey into burger patties.

3. Season the turkey burgers with paprika, garlic powder, and salt.

4. Grill the turkey burgers for about 6-7 minutes per side or until cooked through.

5. While the burgers are cooking, toss sweet potato fries in olive oil and season with paprika and salt.

6. Spread the sweet potato fries on a baking sheet lined with parchment paper and bake in the oven at 425°F (220°C) for about 20-25 minutes or until crispy.

7. Serve the turkey burgers in whole-grain buns or lettuce wraps with your choice of toppings, alongside the sweet potato fries.

Cooking Time: 30 minutes

Fibromyalgia Diet Snacks Recipes

1. Greek Yogurt Parfait

A simple and delicious snack featuring Greek yogurt, granola, and fresh berries for a balanced and nutritious treat.

Ingredients:

- 1/2 cup Greek yogurt
- 1/4 cup granola
- 1/4 cup mixed berries (e.g., strawberries, blueberries)
- Drizzle of honey (optional)

Instructions:

1. In a glass or bowl, layer Greek yogurt, granola, and mixed berries.

2. Drizzle with honey if desired.

3. Repeat layers if desired.

4. Serve chilled.

Cooking Time: 5 minutes

2. Sliced Apple with Almond Butter

A satisfying and energy-boosting snack featuring sliced apples and almond butter.

Ingredients:

- 1 apple, sliced
- 2 tbsp almond butter

Instructions:

1. Slice the apple into wedges.

2. Serve with almond butter for dipping.

Cooking Time: 5 minutes

3. Carrot and Hummus

A crunchy and fiber-rich snack featuring baby carrots and hummus.

Ingredients:

- Baby carrots
- Hummus

Instructions:

1. Wash and prep baby carrots.

2. Serve with hummus for dipping.

Cooking Time: No cooking required

4. Trail Mix

A customizable trail mix featuring a variety of nuts, seeds, and dried fruits for a quick and energizing snack.

Ingredients:

- Almonds
- Walnuts
- Pumpkin seeds
- Dried cranberries
- Raisins
- Dark chocolate chips (optional)

Instructions:

1. Mix all the ingredients together in a bowl.

2. Portion into snack-sized bags for easy, on-the-go snacking.

Cooking Time: No cooking required

5. Rice Cakes with Avocado

A light and creamy snack featuring rice cakes topped with avocado slices.

Ingredients:

- Rice cakes
- 1/2 ripe avocado, sliced
- Salt and pepper to taste

Instructions:

1. Top rice cakes with avocado slices.

2. Season with salt and pepper to taste.

Cooking Time: No cooking required

6. Smoothie with Spinach and Berries

A nutrient-packed green smoothie featuring spinach, mixed berries, and almond milk.

Ingredients:

- Handful of fresh spinach
- 1/2 cup mixed berries (e.g., strawberries, blueberries)
- 1 cup almond milk
- 1 tbsp honey (optional)

Instructions:

1. Blend spinach, mixed berries, and almond milk until smooth.

2. Add honey if desired for sweetness.

3. Pour into a glass and enjoy!

Cooking Time: 5 minutes

7. Cottage Cheese with Pineapple

A protein-rich and sweet snack featuring cottage cheese and fresh pineapple chunks.

Ingredients:

- 1/2 cup cottage cheese
- 1/2 cup fresh pineapple chunks

Instructions:

1. Spoon cottage cheese into a bowl.

2. Top with fresh pineapple chunks.

3. Enjoy this sweet and savory combination.

Cooking Time: No cooking required

8. Homemade Energy Balls

Customizable energy balls made with wholesome ingredients for a quick and satisfying snack.

Ingredients:

- 1 cup rolled oats
- 1/2 cup nut butter (e.g., almond, peanut)

- 1/4 cup honey or maple syrup

- 1/4 cup ground flaxseeds

- 1/4 cup dark chocolate chips (optional)

- 1/4 cup dried fruits (e.g., raisins, apricots)

Instructions:

1. In a bowl, mix together rolled oats, nut butter, honey or maple syrup, ground flaxseeds, dark chocolate chips (if using), and dried fruits.

2. Roll the mixture into bite-sized balls.

3. Place in the refrigerator to set for at least 30 minutes.

4. Store in an airtight container for convenient snacking.

Cooking Time: 30 minutes (mostly inactive)

9. Rice Cake with Cottage Cheese and Berries

A light and creamy snack featuring rice cakes, cottage cheese, and fresh berries.

Ingredients:

- Rice cakes

- 1/2 cup cottage cheese

- 1/4 cup mixed berries (e.g., raspberries, blueberries)

Instructions:

1. Spread cottage cheese onto rice cakes.

2. Top with mixed berries.

Cooking Time: No cooking required

10. Veggie Sticks with Tzatziki Sauce

A crunchy and refreshing snack featuring sliced bell peppers, cucumber, and carrot sticks with tzatziki sauce for dipping.

Ingredients:

- Sliced bell peppers
- Sliced cucumber
- Carrot sticks
- Tzatziki sauce

Instructions:

1. Wash and prep the vegetables.

2. Serve with tzatziki sauce for dipping.

Cooking Time: No cooking required

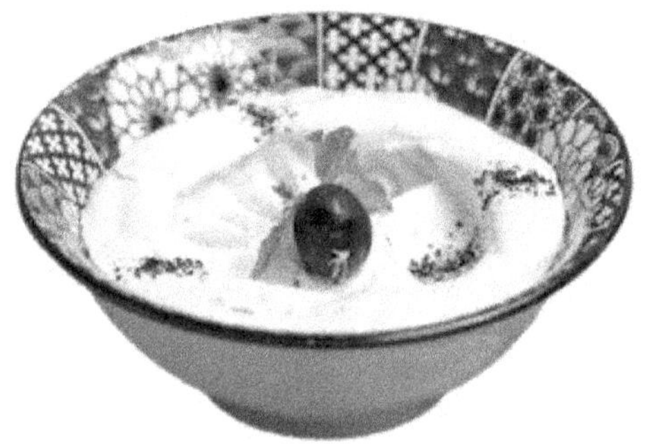

CONCLUSION

The role of diet in managing fibromyalgia cannot be overstated. While there is no one-size-fits-all approach, a well-balanced and carefully chosen diet can significantly impact the quality of life for individuals living with fibromyalgia.

Understanding the types, causes, and symptoms of fibromyalgia is essential for tailoring a diet that suits individual needs. By incorporating foods that are anti-inflammatory, rich in antioxidants, and low in triggers like processed sugars and certain additives, many individuals with fibromyalgia have reported improvements in their symptoms.

The fibromyalgia diet often includes nutrient-dense options such as fruits, vegetables, lean proteins, and whole grains. Omega-3 fatty acids from sources like fatty fish and flaxseeds can help reduce inflammation, while magnesium-rich foods like spinach and almonds may assist in muscle relaxation and pain management.

Moreover, maintaining hydration is crucial, as dehydration can exacerbate symptoms. Balancing macronutrients is equally important, as the right mix of carbohydrates, proteins, and fats can help stabilize energy levels and minimize the severity of fatigue, a common complaint among fibromyalgia sufferers.

Smaller, frequent meals can also aid in maintaining steady energy levels throughout the day. Supplements, under the guidance of a healthcare provider, may be recommended to address specific nutritional deficiencies commonly found in individuals with fibromyalgia, such as vitamin D or magnesium.

It's important to note that dietary changes alone may not provide a complete solution for fibromyalgia management. They are most effective when integrated into a comprehensive treatment plan that includes physical activity, stress management, and medication, if necessary. Always consult with a healthcare provider or registered dietitian before making significant dietary changes to ensure they align with individual health needs and goals.

In conclusion, while there is no cure for fibromyalgia, a thoughtfully designed diet can play a pivotal role in alleviating symptoms and improving overall well-being. By embracing a fibromyalgia-friendly diet and making informed choices, individuals can take proactive steps toward enhancing their quality of life and achieving better symptom management.